My Journey on Losing 10kg in 12 Months.

Bonita Gonsalvez

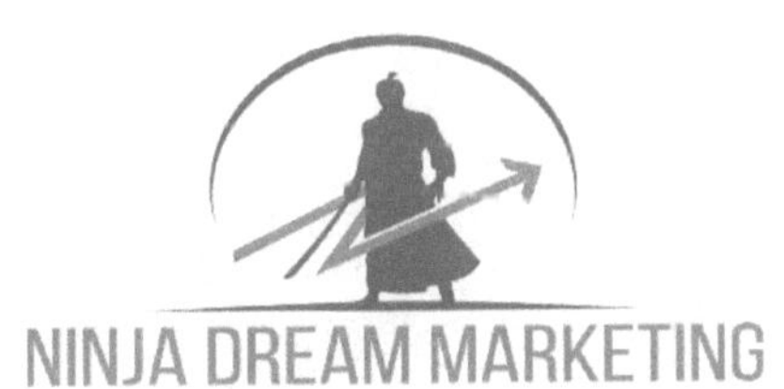

<u>**FREE**</u> **OFFER!**
5 Easy Keto recipes to get you started on your journey to weight loss

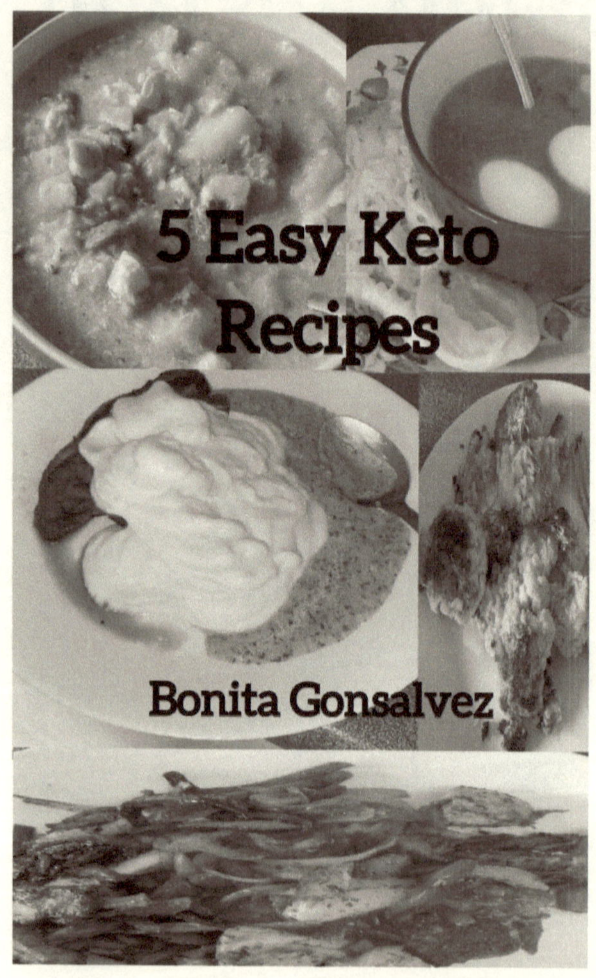

https://www.ninjadreammarketing.com/FREEeasyketorecipes

Disclaimer Page

Dedication

I would like to dedicate this book to everyone who is struggling to lose weight. This is dedicated to supporting you on your journey to weight loss.

Contents

Acknowledgements

I would like to thank my friends, family, fitness advisors, teachers, supervisors, and mentors for all their support and motivation on my journey to weight loss.

1.About me and my struggle with weight loss

Hi, my name is Bonita Gonsalvez. I work in the healthcare sector and have always struggled to lose weight during several stages of my life. All in all, this impacted my health and the relationships I had with various people. After a lot of trial and error, I have made changes about myself and lost approximately 10kg in 12 months. I aim to help other people like me to get into a better place mentally, physically, and emotionally. In this report, I describe the challenges that I faced and the various changes that I made to feel good about myself and my body.

2.My journey towards weight loss

So, after weighing myself on my scales, I realised that I needed to do something about my weight as it was getting ridiculous. This is what I thought to myself, "Bonita, if you do not take actions and steps now, your weight will just increase. You will just feel chubby, big, and bloated. NOW is the time to take action". I had enough of those voices nagging at me all the time, so I joined a local gym and followed a personal trainer's initial advice. I was lucky that the gym offered a three-week induction for free. There, the personal trainer made a three-week plan for me and I followed the plan from beginning to end. I gained some motivation and ideas on the regimes/workouts that I should be doing to carry on with my journey to weight loss. Unfortunately, I did not have the finances to afford a personal trainer. So, I had to look for other options that were much cheaper than a monthly/weekly recurring bill in addition to my gym membership. I started to look for a weight loss programme online and came across a 3-month fitness programme for the one-time payment of $99. I listened to the instructors and watched their videos. I then followed their exercise routines and paid close attention to the emphasis of their exercise.

My exercise programme was as follows:
1. Cardiovascular training.
2. Resistance training

Cardiovascular training

Cardiovascular training is a tool for aerobic fitness to increase the oxygen uptake that reaches the tissues in our body. Aerobic exercise primarily involves the movement of large muscle groups. Exercises include jogging, running, biking, and swimming. Cardiovascular is essential for weight loss. I followed a 3-6 week plan of cardiovascular exercise with advisors from my local gym. I also performed some exercises for resistance training.

Resistance training

Muscular fitness is done through resistance training. Resistance training is achieved through:

1. Bodyweight
2. Weights
3. Machines

I followed a 3-month fitness programme which included resistance training and during my journey to weight loss, I performed some research to find out how I could maximise my efforts and optimise my weight loss. So, I invested in supplements, bought branched-chain amino acid (BCAAS), creatinine, pre-workout and post-workout powders. As I followed the exercise programme and took some enhancements, I lost 10 kg in 12 months. Now, this was not easy. I had some changes to make regarding my mindset and motivations and had to identify factors that were influencing my progress to weight loss.

3.The challenges that I faced during my journey to weight loss:

Everyone in your friends, family, and work circles seem to be against you and your new habits. As I started my journey to weight loss, I realised that the habits that online experts describe are very different from that of my family and colleagues. My new habits became obvious to others and they started to show their concerns about my new habits and some commented that I should be following their way of living. My advice on this is to look at the people you are talking to and see if they are qualified or have experience/ have done the work to get a good and functioning body or have a healthy lifestyle. To overcome this, identify the individuals that are likely to have a negative mindset so that you become more aware and can control all the conflicts associated with their mindset. I joined a weight loss support network on a Facebook group where I know that there are like-minded individuals and experts that could guide me through making the right steps for weight loss. Other like-minded individuals have joined local meetings that specialise in weight loss. If you do this, it will make you feel that the steps that you have taken are correct and help you improve your habits.

Motivation and Mindset

Sometimes, you will have individuals (experts) pushing you to one extreme and throwing words or workouts at you that you may not be comfortable with and may not be aware of. It is important to realise that these individuals are doing this to push you to your best but if there are workouts that you do not enjoy, then please point this out to the individuals concerned. Exercises can be made and designed so that you enjoy what you do and feel motivated to carry on doing the work to improve your fitness. Therefore, it is important to choose individuals that you feel you can work with and can keep you motivated to do the work for your fitness. If you are dreading the course or the personal trainer, then this is a sign that perhaps this may not be the right personal trainer or course for you and most importantly, just remember that you have the option to change it!

S.M.A.R.T goals

My goals were set with experts and they were S.M.A.R.T (Specific, Measurable, Realistic and Tangible). I just knew my BMI was outside the range and just wanted it to be within the norm. I told them what my ideal weight was. I didn't care how and when but I just wanted to improve my health. If you cannot set SMART goals for yourself, then find someone that can do this for you for starters. Perhaps they can help you construct one so you know what you are aiming for subconsciously. Most importantly, surround yourself with individuals that can advise you properly.

4.What did I change about myself?

Mindset

My mindset has changed, and it has influenced people around me. One of my personal experiences on how your growth mindset is different from that of others during my journey to weight loss will be described with a basic fact on weight loss and an example of my experience. When you are on a journey to lose weight, you must drink more water. The amount of water you drink depends on your body weight. You should do your research to find out how much you should be drinking during your journey. The example is that people at my workplace started putting pressure on me when I started to drink more water to hydrate my body because I was going to the bathroom more than usual. Luckily, I did my research and found out that this transition is perfectly normal. The moral of the story is that you do indeed have to change the way you think and surround yourself with experts or like-minded individuals to persevere and achieve the results that you want. This may or may not apply to you. It depends on your surroundings and socio-economic impact. Once you start doing the work, you will notice

that you influence others and their unhealthy habits.
Because of my new mindset and ability to challenge
my colleagues, they started to hydrate themselves
more often. I must admit, I did not enjoy having to
justify myself for making a healthy change in my life.
Hopefully, this book will help you identify those
individuals and will not deter you from making progress

Diet

I have researched and paid for meal plans that could help me in the process of losing weight. They can be as cheap as $45-50. If you start and follow through with it, I am sure that the way you once looked at food will change. If you are anxious about going for a plan or diet right from the start, then I recommend that you start with the very basics.

Things to look at:

1. How much am I eating?
2. Can I reduce my portions?
3. Can I introduce more fruits or vegetables into my diet?
4. Can I improve what I am eating with minor changes until

I feel ready to push myself to the next level?

For my personal experience, I started to do some exercises to make myself feel better. The science behind it is, the more you exercise, the more you release happy chemicals called endorphins. As I became happier, I was able to focus. The voices that were in my head had gone as I implemented something and stuck to it until I received results. And if I did not, I found a way to overcome it myself or asked for help from experts. Once I had improved my fitness and gained confidence, I started to follow a ketogenic diet.

5.Keto Diet

A keto diet is where you restrict yourself from eating carbohydrates. Traditionally, in school, we are taught to follow the food triangle and are convinced that our diet should have a huge proportion of carbohydrates. In a ketogenic diet, we are trying to make our body burn fat. We restrict the amount of carbohydrate we eat and opt for a higher proportion of vegetables and salad. After switching to a ketogenic diet, I felt energised, less moody lost some kilos and improved my cooking skills. I am also gaining ideas to cook accompanied by smoothies. There are plenty of ketogenic recipes, plans, and smoothies. Pick a meal plan and stick with it. You will improve over time

6.My next steps:

As I began to solve one big problem in my life, I realised that there will always be other problems and challenges that come along, whether they are personal or fitness. Once you have achieved a specific goal, there will be yet another goal to achieve. You need to keep going after each hurdle and challenge. My next step is to look for other programmes that can help me lose more weight as by now, I have gained muscle through my 3-month training programme. So, I can look at other programmes that can optimise my journey to weight loss and perhaps change my current meals. You will notice that your diet and exercise will keep changing during your journey to weight loss. This is perfectly normal as each workout and programme focuses on different goals for you to achieve your ultimate goal which is to lose weight. For example, you may not be able to withstand the original programme that was designed to enable you to lose weight because of fats, your body shape or any medical conditions which you might have. Therefore, you would need to follow some other programme that can prepare your body for the programme which was designed for you to lose weight. I can confirm this as I was not able to perform some push-ups due to my body weight, body shape, and fats all over my body. So, I had to do some muscle training to perform push-ups and burn fat effectively. If you ask for a consultation with an expert, they will be able to guide you and create a plan suited to you, your body and any condition that you may have. Please do not compare your plan or body to others if you plan to lose weight with friends. Just remember that everyone's body, structure, and conditions are different.

7.Conclusion:

In summary, if you have the willpower and motivation to lose weight, you will achieve what you are looking for. The main point of this report is for you to learn who can influence the way you think about your lifestyle and how you can change it by joining a community or support group and explore the various options that are available for you to achieve your goals. As always, do not compare yourself to others. You can control your thoughts and your journey to weight loss. Do whatever it takes to overcome your obstacles! I hope that this report motivates you to take steps to improve your health

About the Author

Bonita Gonsalvez moved from a small tropical island called Mauritius and settled down in the United Kingdom with her family. From a young age, she was bullied for being obese and has always struggled with weight loss despite making several attempts to lose fat. This affected her mental health and her relationships with people. Over the past year, Bonita has implemented several changes to her mindset and her life and has successfully lost 10kg. She has identified factors that previously inhibited her progress to weight loss and found ways to overcome them. In this book, she shares her personal experience of losing fat and dropping the kilos. Her mindset has been reset and she is currently looking for ways to further improve her health.

She originally trained as a scientist at Cambridge University Hospital, United Kingdom and studied for a BSc and MSc in Colchester. She used her reading, writing and research skills to complete research work at a research institute in London. Her interests lie in writing books for entertainment and that aim to improve peoples' lives

Reviews

Dear Reader,

I hope this book motivates you to start your journey to weight loss. I wrote this book to help people who were struggling to lose weight and help them identify any factors within their environment that may be impeding their progress. While this isn't the perfect formula, hopefully it can give you an idea to get started and prevent these factors from interfering with your progress to weight reduction. Hopefully, you can find ways to make it work for you.
Finally, if you have time, I'd really love a review. Reviews are huge help to authors. I would appreciate your feedback. Love it or hate it, a detailed feedback will help make my work better. If you have time, here's a link to my author page: amazon.com/author/bonitagonsalvez

Other books by Bonita Gonsalvez:

This is Bonita's first book. Previously, she built her audience by writing reports and essays during her career as a scientist. She has engaged with researchers on Research Gate and listened to their feedback to improve her writing skills. Therefore, this is her first publication with Amazon. Bonita is extremely passionate about her writing and wants to provide useful information for her audience to act and improve their lives, just as she has. Equally, in the future, she plans to write books for entertainment. "My Journey on Losing 10kg in 12 Months " is based around Bonita's personal experience.

Ketogenic Food

(Bonita's diet experience)

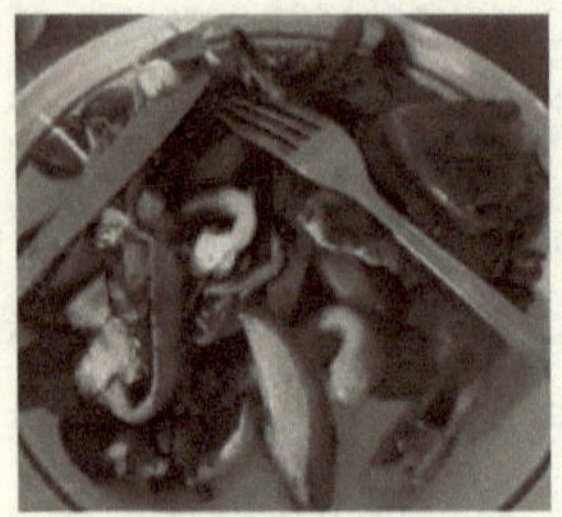

Lamb with Peppers and salad

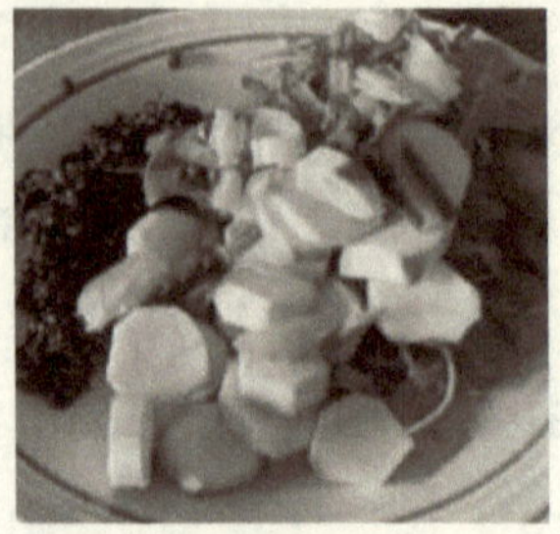

Minced lamb in tamarind sauce with zucchini and salad

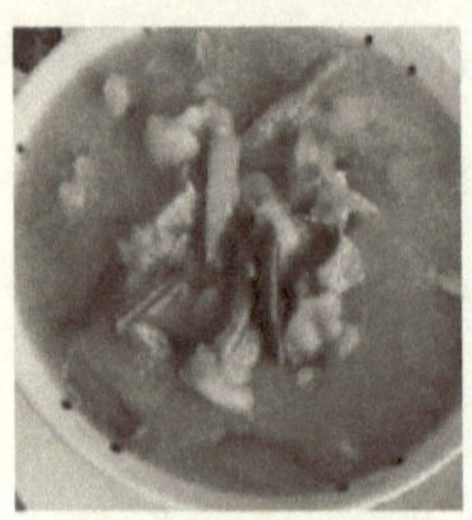

Lamb soup with vegetables

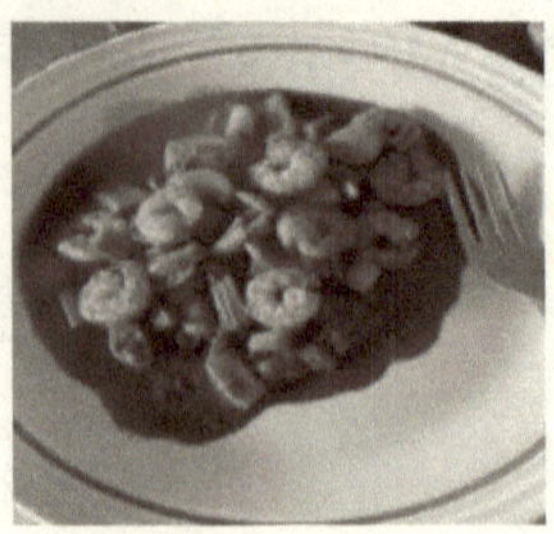

Prawn Curry

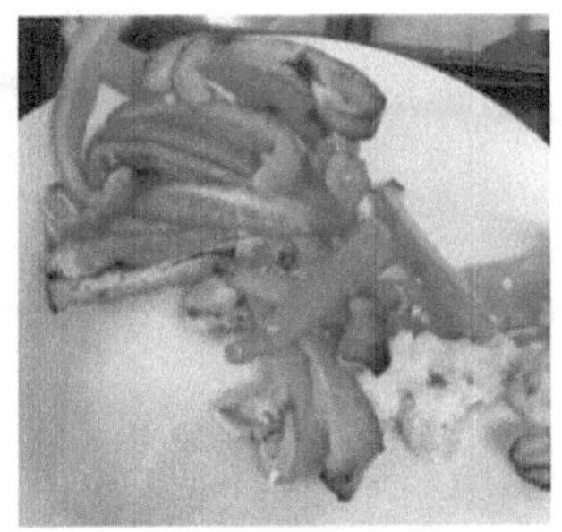

Roast Garlic chicken and Peppers

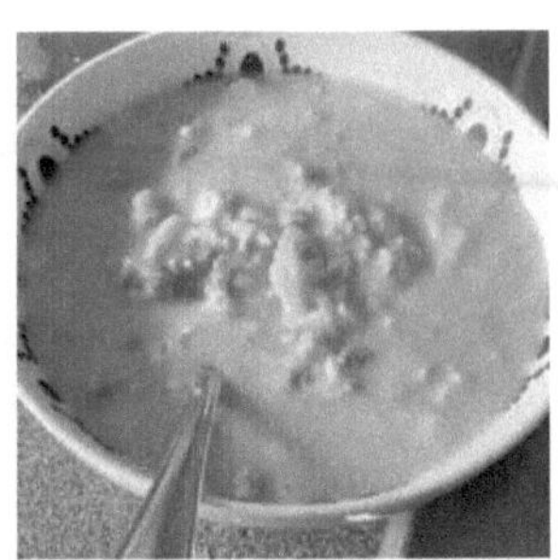

Minced lamb soup with ginger

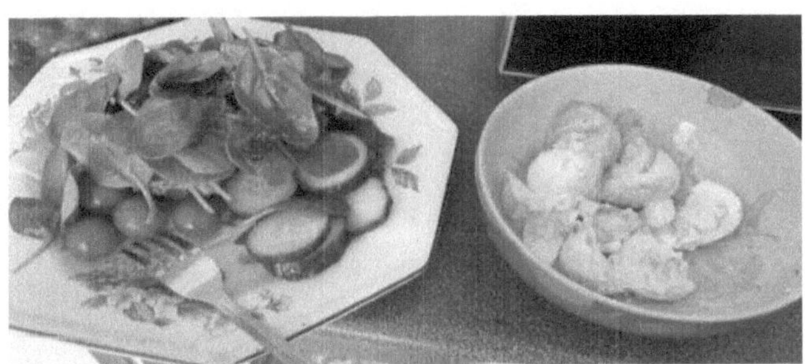

Egg in mustard with salad

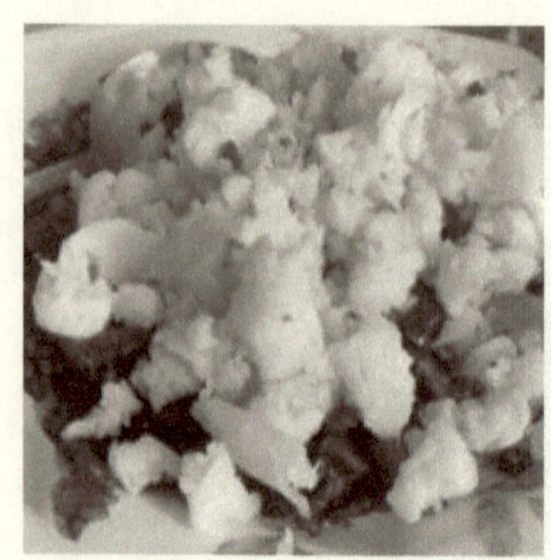

Lamb steak with Cauliflower rice

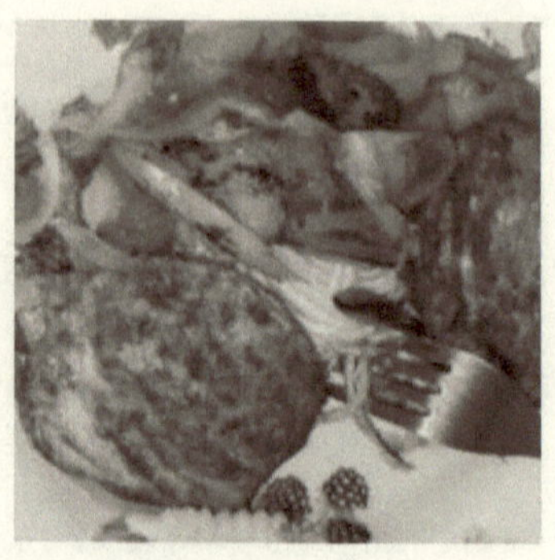

Minced lamb patties, zucchini noodles, onion and tomato sauce

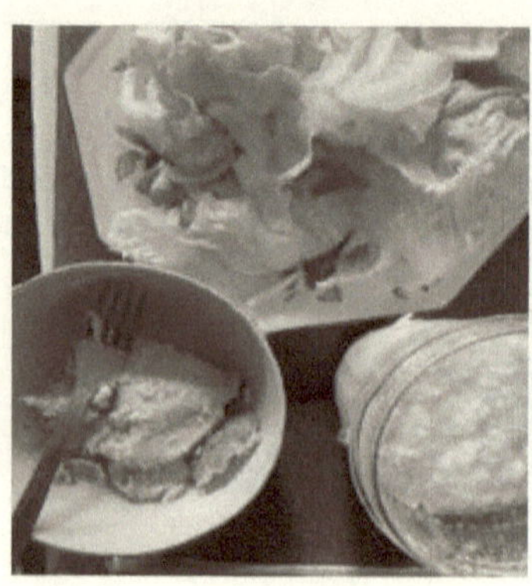

Macadamian coated chicken with salad and lemon smoothie

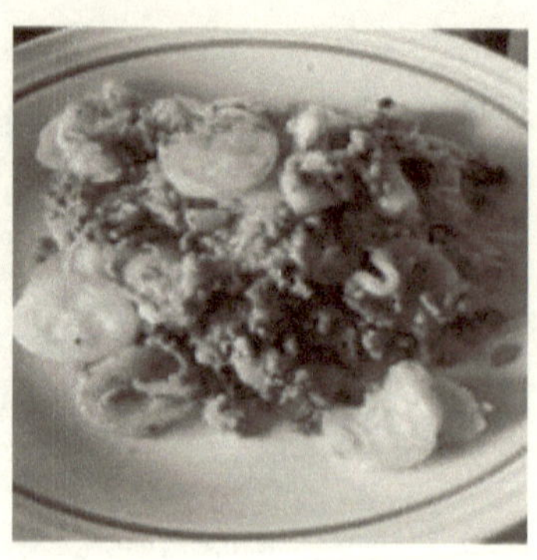

Minced lamb with Zucchini noodles

Join us for FREE

Keep up to date with Bonita's diet:

https://www.instagram.com/wealthyandhealthyliving/

Company social media links:

Our company page:
https://www.facebook.com/ninjadreammarketingltd

Our company website:
https://www.ninjadreammarketing.com/

Keep updated with our company on Instagram

https://www.instagram.com/ninjadreammarketingltd/

Keep up to date with us on LinkedIn:
https://www.linkedin.com/company/54113070/admin/

Subscribe to our YouTube channel:
https://www.youtube.com/channel/UC_jiU9nHTOISspJ1JEaHM2g?view_as=subscriber

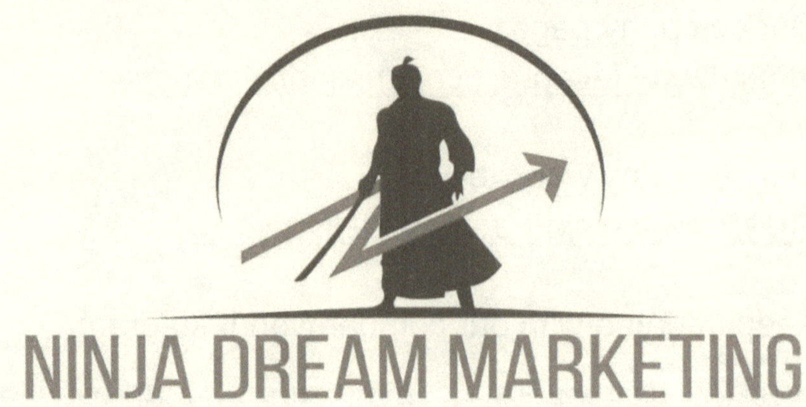

NINJA DREAM MARKETING